I0510892

Bacteriophage Could Be a Hurdle in the Path of Progression of Viral Infection - a Review

Nishat Zafar
Muhammad Aamir Aslam
Syeda Zainab Akhlaq
Muhammad Tariq Javid

ELIVA PRESS

ELIVA PRESS

Nishat Zafar
Muhammad Aamir Aslam
Syeda Zainab Akhlaq
Muhammad Tariq Javid

Literature studies will become essential to check possible known interactions before choosing the contender bacteriophages. For example, it has been shown that when bacteria are exposed to their specific bacteriophages, biofilm produced by some bacteria could create difficulties for virus infected patients in developing treatment methods. Some bacteriophages can live inside the host without harming them while mostly kills their bacterial host. The present study provides many precautions to be followed carefully. For a while, in viral infected patients with severe respiratory failure, complex immune deregulation has been observed. Bacteriophages can be used for treatment because they can be prepared cheaply and quickly when it is probably to prove experimental. Some production values may be shown by antibody production from phage display techniques, but it should be easy or straightforward due to current development. Moreover, bacteriophages can be easy to store and transport. Virus prevalence is diminished by bacteriophages, especially in the patients affected by high viral load and bacterial infection of secondary type because they can be an experimental tool. There are no significant side effects, so it plays a vital role in saving lives. The beauty of nature showed us the mini creature that may be harmful but influential in the other aspects.

Published by Eliva Press SRL

Address: MD-2060, bd.Cuza-Voda, 1/4, of. 21 Chişinău, Republica Moldova

Email: info@elivapress.com

Website: www.elivapress.com

ISBN: 978-1-63648-085-5

Table of Contents

Nishat Zafar[*], Muhammad Aamir Aslam, Syeda Zainab Akhlaq, Muhammad Tariq Javid

Institute of Microbiology, University of Agriculture, Faisalabad, Punjab, Pakistan

*Email: Nishat Zafar

nishat_zafar@yahoo.com

Abstract: The coronavirus disease (Covid-19) pandemic has caused the loss of an estimated 270,000 people as of the 8th of May 2020. This study emphasizes bacteriophages' possible function to minimize the patient's death rate affected by the severe acute respiratory syndrome coronavirus 2 (SARS-CoV-2) virus. The secondary cause of death in Covid-19 is miscommunication between the innate and adaptive immune responses, culminating in the inability to generate successful antibodies to the virus on time. While more study is desperately required, secondary bacterial infections in the respiratory system could ultimately lead to the high mortality rate among older people due to Covid-19. If bacterial development, along with cognitive impairments of antibodies, is a significant contributor to Covid-19's death rates, the increased time required for the human body's adaptive immune capacity to make specific antibodies could be obtained by slowing the levels of bacterial growth in the patient's respiratory system. Independently of that, the use of synthetic antibodies to SARS-CoV-2 viruses could substantially reduce the infection rate. Decreased microbial population and covalent binding of synthetic antibodies to viruses should further influence the concentration of inflammatory fluids in patients' lungs. While antibiotics may theoretically accomplish the first target, I suggest that other approaches could be more efficient or used in conjunction with antibiotics to suppress bacteria's growth rate and that the corresponding clinical studies should be undertaken. The bacterial inflation rate could theoretically be decreased by using natural bacteriophage aerosols to feed on the major species of bacteria believed to cause respiratory distress and be hazardous to the patient. Independently of this, synthetically engineered bacteriophages could be used for the rapid production of particular antibodies to SARS-CoV-2. This can be achieved using a Nobel Prize-winning procedure called 'phage show.' If it succeeds, the patient is given additional time to generate their particular antibodies to the SARS-CoV-2 virus and avoid the damage caused by an extreme immunological reaction.

INTRODUCTION

Promptly spread of SARS-CoV-2 (Severe Acute Respiratory Syndrome Coronavirus 2) pandemic is currently being faced by the world, which causes COVID-19 disease (Sung, 2004). World Health Organization reported more than 270,000 deaths by 8th May 2020, and the coronavirus pandemic was responsible for these casualties. In Covid-19, one of the most dangerous symptoms that we observe is the properties of this virus (SARS-Cov-2) and the combined effect of globalization, which causes the Severe Acute Respiratory Syndrome Coronavirus 2. Although this respiratory attacking virus warns of the threat of long-term pose and consistency globally, it also devastates the economy's infrastructure and health. Multiple and urgent approaches need to

3

tackle this problem (Cevik et al., 2020).

There are many candidates at the time of writing in the pipeline to fight against coronavirus that claims many promising treatments and vaccine-like Pfizer's coronavirus vaccine. (Huang et al. 2020) However, at the time, there are no specific treatments or vaccines available for COVID-19. This deadly nature of disease creates many challenges in different areas such as government policies, public health, and more on the world's economy by posing unprecedented effects (Maslov and Sneppen, 2017). Observations on other conditions such as HIV, malaria, and tuberculosis over the last few decades have shown that the pandemic's solution without vaccination or treatment requires multifaceted and useful measurements. (Tay et al., 2020)

On the other hand, highly effective and efficient vaccines have proven for plenty of diseases such as nascent influenza to control and prevent their spread. Unfortunately, the underdeveloped vaccine's efficiency and productivity to prevent and limit the spread of SARS-CoV-2 is still unknown. Furthermore, in severe cases or patients with different diseases and other health conditions, there may be additional treatments to develop, even if the first vaccine or therapy is successful for any candidate. (Shi and Gewirtz, 2018) In drug development, bacteriophages can play an essential role in controlling or limiting the COVID-19 pandemic as a potential approach to find the leads, and this editorial focuses on it. (Stiasny et al. 2012)

Potential Importance of Bacteria in the Development of Symptoms for Covid-19

The respiratory system is the most feasible route used by SARS-CoV-2 to enter the human body. After entering the human body, the virus disrupts the respiratory system's stability (Ventura et al., 2017). Miscommunication between adaptive and innate immune responses may be an unintended cause of death in patients suffering from Covid-19. To attack a pathogen efficiently, adaptive immune responses are required much more time than innate immune responses. This implies that a moment comes when the only fighter against the virus is natural immunity as innate immunity has to deal with the increased load of virus alone, affecting other body systems. (Grijalva et al., 2014) As the virus grows and multiplies in the lungs, the natural immune system begins to secrete fluids and cells, which cause inflammation of the lungs. It leads to a low exchange of gases as the lungs are occupied with inflammatory fluid. (Butler and Schuchat, 1999)

Respiratory cells of humans infected with the virus and died can become a source of food for bacteria and allow it to grow. It is one of the side effects of viral infection. Bacterial growth triggers more innate immune responses. (Almand et al., 2017) As a result, more inflammatory fluid is secreted in neighboring alveoli. In this way, bacterial infection facilitates viral infection by aggravating more innate immune responses. This process continues, and more respiratory cells become infected and killed by the virus. This cell debris further initiates bacterial growth. Bacterial growth trigger different innate immune responses and more inflammatory fluid are secreted in the lungs. (Bosch et al., 2013) Then a moment comes when the lungs are occupied with the provocative fluid hindering exchange of gases. It may result in septic shock and death. So ventilators are immediately required.

In older people, SARS-CoV-2 is riskier because virus-specific antibodies either do not produce or produced later. (Zhou et al., 2020) Immunity against Covid-19 is currently reviewed in detail, and According to a current review that completely describes the latest information about immune responses against the Covid-19 virus, this disease progresses differently in old and young people. (Dagur, 2020)

Delayed production of virus-specific antibodies is mainly due to damage to immune functions (Immunosenescence), and it is commonly observed in aged people. This may be why the high death rate due to Covid-19 in older people (Langan et al., 2015). There is limited data available on Covid-19, but it is concluded from facts that a person who has previously suffered from influenza is more prone to pneumococcal colonization. So, a well-known mechanism exists which is used by the virus to cause pulmonary infection of bacteria. (Seki et al., 2004)

Moreover, besides the Covid-19 virus, other viruses also cause bacterial infections (the detailed mechanism of COVID-19 is shown in Figure 1). Succession is a term used by ecologists, and secondary infection is a term used by medical doctors for this co-existence of bacteria and virus. In the patients suffering from influenza, *Staphylococcus aureus*, *Aerococcus viridans, Staphylococcus pneumonia, Moraxella catarrhalis Haemophilus influenza,* and other bacteria which are part of the normal flora of the respiratory tract also co-exist with the influenza virus. Sometimes, these bacteria are converted into pathogenic bacteria and cause infection. (Radetsky, 1994)

A current review proposes that bacterial infections caused by *Klebsiella pneumonia* and *Acinetobacter baumanii* have been recognized in patients suffering from Covid-19, particularly those present in the ICU. Most probably secondary infection and sepsis, but results regarding the detailed study of bacteria were not mentioned. Steroids also enhance the chances of secondary infection to occur. (Al-Shayeb, 2020)

The bacterial infection might contribute to a small proportion of death associated with Covid-19, but the exact number is not assessed. It might be challenging to determine a precise number because of the large number of Covid-19 patients in clinics, standard measures for which they come to the lab for bacteriology testing, and the state at which disease progresses. (Shkoporov and Hill, 2019) It has been currently reported from Wuhan that secondary infection was observed in 50% of patients who died of Covid-19. On average, 17 days are required to develop secondary infections, though the time range is extended. It is acceptable that bacteria start to colonize the respiratory tract before developing acute respiratory distress syndrome. (Koskella and Meaden., 2013)

In the case of influenza, infection of *Pseudomonas aeruginosa* spreads very quickly. Furthermore, massive and quick response of the innate immune system (first line of defense) leads to inflammation, which causes fibrosis (alteration of pulmonary structure). As a result, uptake of oxygen is further decreased, which damages pulmonary tissues permanently. In this case, the innate immune system is responsible for the death. Nevertheless, the degree to which the natural immune system responds to SARS-CoV-2 or bacterial infection like pseudomonas aeruginosa infection is still unknown and different during disease progression. (Mueller, 1973) The relation between the human body's period to produce antibodies against the Covid-19 virus and aged people's death due to bacterial infection is still unknown.

There are many disadvantages to using antibiotics. One drawback is that antibiotics kill both beneficial and harmful bacteria, but phages kill only harmful bacteria. Moreover, misuse of antibiotics leads to the development of resistance to antibiotics and produces ''superbugs'' (bacteria that become immune to antibiotics). (Papkou et al., 2019)

During the current pandemic of Covid-19, antibiotics are given to 70% of COVID-19 patients present in hospitals worldwide. It enhances the risk of the development of antibiotic-resistance in bacteria. (Willing et al., 2012) More strategies are required as an alternative to antibiotics to control the infections caused by antibiotic-resistant bacteria. Contrary to antibiotics, bacteriophages significantly reduce the chances of the emergence of resistance because they acclimatize to prevent antibiotic resistance in bacteria. (Salyers, 2003)

Proposal of Integrative Methodology
The growth of bacteria and the delay in antibody production contribute significantly to the death rate due to the Covid-19 virus. For adaptive immunity to produce virus-specific antibodies, additional time is required. (Aslam, 2018) If the quality of bacterial growth in the respiratory system is decreased, this extra time can be quickly gained. This reduced bacterial growth should lead to a reduced rate at which liquid is filled in the lungs. Nevertheless, if the viral growth rate is high, it should also be reduced to decrease the rate of immune responses. (Hsu, 2020)

History of Bacteriophage
According to Summer et al., bacteriophage history could be divided into four timespans.

Early Enthusiasm
In 1915, Twort, an English microbiologist, was discovered bacteriophages, but in 1917, French-Canadian microbiologist Felix d' Herelle performed experiments on bacteriophages. Firstly, he tested the safety of bacteriophages on himself by injected and ingested and became successful. During his experiments, he saw some microscopic organisms in the stool filtrate of dysentery patients and

observed that they were antagonist to bacteria (Pelfrene et al., 2017). He concluded that this filterable microorganism was acted as a cofactor of bacterial infection. After his successful experiments, in 1919, he treated patients suffering from cholera and bacillary dysentery and then wound healing (Prazak et al., 2019). In 1926, avian typhosis was caused by *Salmonella gallinarum,* and *Pasteurella multocida* was an infectious agent of bovine hemorrhagic septicemia; scientists investigated the healing ability of bacteriophages against these diseases. These trials also confirmed the protection of phages. However, Bruynoghe and Maisin work was described as phage therapy, and its results were published in 1921 (Summers, 2010).

Critical Scepticism

Even though, in earlier several trials against bacteriophage therapy, positive results and dissatisfaction were also revealed. In a report, previously released data were criticized, which was published in 1934 (Merrill et al., 2016). According to the researchers, the phage nature, strengths, and limitations were not well known. However, some mistakes were shown in the report, as the lack of standard protocol in preparing phages, and there were no principles to compare the experimentation results (Miedzybrodzki et al., 2007).

Abandonment

In the USA, the research on bacteriophages was reversed away due to the discovery of antibiotics. The ease of production, broad range activity and stability in the preparation process were the benefits of using antibiotics compared to bacteriophage therapy (Golkar et al., n.d.). The two military-based countries in Europe, such as Germany and the Soviet Union, used bacteriophages to treat wound healing. In the Soviet Union, phage applications were mostly economic and ideational motives ("preponderance" of Soviet science over the capitalist West). However, through D'Herelle, Georgia founded the State Serum and Vaccine Institute in Tbilisi, one of the foremost bacteriophage therapy centers (Bonilla et al., 2016). The curious fact of phage therapy is that the Pasteur institute where d'Herelle worked on bacteriophages, also known as the mother institute of d'Herelle, got their phages mostly from Georgia and Russia, even at present (Abedon & Thomas-abedon, 2010). One more reason for ending the era of bacterial viruses was developing resistance against bacteriophages. Another problem is the unwittingness of pathogenic bacteria's mechanism and the nature of the association between phage and its host (Chaudhry et al., 2013).

Recent Interest and Reappraisal

In Pakistan, several experiments using phage therapy against cholera infection were funded by WHO in the 1970s (Caprinos, 2008). The deduction of these reports could be a proclamation that phage therapy against cholera infection is not an effective means of treatment than tetracycline antibiotic treatment (Klumpp et al., 2010). Moreover, phages against cholera infection can specifically diminish the vibrios population without affecting the microflora and no visible side effects on the patients. Hence, phage therapy might be a useful study tool. Some other articles showed that phage therapy treated diarrheal infection caused by Escherichia coli in the lab and farm animals (Lu & Koeris, 2011). It is concluded that phages could be applied in medical treatment and prophylaxis. These researches were commenced the bacteriophage recovery, driven by the rich trove of Soviet and Polish work. Study in Poland has been conducted mostly on thousands of patients in association with the Hirszfeld institute of Immunology and experimental therapy in Wroclaw (Fadlallah et al., 2015). Likewise, all these studies were believed to be most accurately documented. In the entire history of phage therapy, thousands of experiments have been performed and involved many other etiologic factors of infections of humans, animals, and microorganisms such as *Acinetobacter, Burkholderia, Salmonella, Citrobacter, Enterobacter, Enterococcus, Proteus, Pseudomonas, Shigella, Staphylococcus, and Streptococcus* (Aminov et al., 2010).

How Do Bacteriophages Kill Bacteria?
The growing rate of a multidrug-resistant strain of bacteria is a significant health issue in modern age medication. Lytic phages can kill the number of multidrug-resistant strains on the completion of the bacteriophage infection cycle (Valleys et al., 2015). Mainly bacteriophages have two lytic mechanisms that can destroy the bacteria's cell wall to release phage progeny successfully. Thus the use of bacteriophage therapy is a potential tool to treat bacterial diseases (Abedon et al., 2011). The phage infection cycle is divided into two stages: lytic and lysogenic processes—the lysis of the bacterial cell required to release lytic phage progeny from the infected cell. Many lytic phages have a single protein known as amurins, which helps inhibit the synthesis of peptidoglycan (Gill & Hyman, 2010).

Moreover bacteriophages used two sets of proteins to kill the bacterial cell. The first is the holin enzymes, and the second one is the endolysin enzymes. Holin is made up of the association with endolysins and is called holin lysin systems (Meyer et al., 2013). Holin caused the triggering process in the host cell, which involved the perforation of the bacterial cytoplasmic membrane and, hence, associated with the enzyme endolysin, which gives entry to the bacteria's peptidoglycan. Hence holin enzymes regulate the lysis of bacterial cells because

11

they control the accessibility of bacterial murein for endolysin enzymes (Kutter et al., 2015). Therefore, they synchronize the holin lysin system's mechanism with the events of the late phage replication cycle. Holin's primary structure is not well known, and its function does not reflect variation in amino acid sequences (Pirnay et al., 2011). Every single holin enzyme has one hydrophobic transmembrane region and a C-terminal hydrophilic region containing a high electric charge. Holin is classified into three classes, such as Class I, Class II, and Class III. Class I containing proteins have a minimum of 95 residues of amino acid in length and three TMDs (Pirnay et al., 2015). So, Staphylococcus aureus phage p68 hol15 protein and E. coli bacteriophage k S105 protein are Class I. Classes II of holin enzymes containing 65-95 residues of amino acid in length (Ryan et al., 2011). These holin enzymes have two TMDs. Class II is characterized by Lambdoid phage 21 S protein and Clostridium perfringens bacteriophage A3626 hol3626 protein (Plaza et al., 2018).

Classes III have only one TMD and are characterized by the phage ACP26F holin S105. This type of phage confines in the cell membrane, and after a precise time point, it can make pathogenic lesions or holes in the lipid bilayer structure of the plasma membrane. These holes have more than 340nm in diameter. Endolysins enzymes of bacteriophages are involved in the degradation of the bacterial cell wall (Rakonjac & Bennett, 2009). Sometimes, they act as a murein degrader to kill bacteria through some enzymes such as endopeptidase, amidase, glycosidase, and lytic transglycosylase (Chan et al., 2013).

Endolysin endorse the release of phage progeny at the end of the replication cycle. The mechanism of action of endolysin against gram-negative bacteria is usually different from the action against gram-positive bacteria (Drulis-kawa et al., 2012). An outer membrane surrounds the gram-negative bacteria, and thus the entry through the cell wall is restricted. Therefore endolysin has small globular proteins comprised of the enzymatically active domain (EAD), which give access to the cell wall of gram-negative bacteria (Endersen et al., 2014). In contrast to gram-positive bacteria, cell wall binding domain (CBD) are present in the endolysin. When endolysin attacking gram-positive bacteria binds to the cell wall by its region of CBD and then localized on the peptidoglycan's surface (Arndt et al., 2016). The cell wall binding domain gives hydrolytic effects and synergistically with the enzymatically active domain, which performs the cell wall's catalytic activity. During this mechanism, endolysin is immobilized on one side of the peptidoglycan. The holin lysin mechanism contributes to the termination of bacteriophage's infection cycle after a specific time duration (Ryan et al., 2012).

Bacteriophages-Natural Weapon to Control Bacterial Growth
Bacteriophages are viruses that infect specific bacterial species and cause them to lyse. But they do not cause infection in animal and human cells. William Twort and Felix d'Herelle discovered bacteriophages in 1915. Bacteriophages are dispersed worldwide and infect a broad range of bacterial hosts and bacterial species naturally present in the human body. (Czaplewski et al., 2016)

It has been demonstrated that bacteriophages infect specific species even though the particular strain of a species.[19] Specificity of bacteriophages also indicates ''Red Queen'' co-evolutionary process between these two players (bacteriophages and bacteria co-exist). Necessary steps involved in bacteriophage infection of the bacterial cell which includes bacteriophage attaches to specific receptor site present on susceptible bacterial cell, take over the control of host biochemical machinery and produce many copies of the virus, lyses of bacterial host occur to release new bacteriophages which further infect other bacterial species mainly belong to same species. (Blanco-Picazo et al., 2020)

Despite the well-known relation between bacteriophages and bacteria, research on bacteriophages and their therapeutic use has not been done for many years because of the antibiotics revolution. (Nale, 2018) Antibiotics were mainly used for the treatment of infections caused by bacteria. The reason is that antibiotics are used for a general-purpose contrary to bacteriophages, which infect specific species of the bacterial host. Besides these, antibiotics act quickly and efficiently. Moreover, antibiotics are synthesized economically. (Nir-Paz et al., 2019)

It has been proposed that bacteriophages positively affect human health and help the patient to recover soon. It implies that bacteriophages play a role in maintaining the balance of microorganisms. For example, a group found bacteriophages to effectively kill the bacteria while evaluating alternative treatment of Clostridium difficile (the bacteria that cause diarrhea due to infection in the bowel). Nowadays, bacteriophages are used for therapeutic purposes. There are many examples of using bacteriophages as a treatment for animal or human models besides using bacteriophages for recently developed bioengineering strategies. (Cafora et al., 2019)

Bacteriophages Speed up the Synthesis of Anti-viral Antibodies used for Therapy:

Undoubtedly, bacteriophages' therapeutic potential to control bacterial infections has been rediscovered, and Nobel prizes were awarded for using them as molecular tools. Moreover, bacteriophages exhibit the ability to produce recombinant antibodies rapidly by using the phage display technique. (Peng et al., 2020) This recombinant antibody production method was established for MERS- CoV and utilized to control MERS- CoV effectively. Phage display is characterized by using all methods that block the interaction of an enzyme ACE2 (Angiotensin-converting enzyme 2) isolated from the serum of patients who become immune to infection. (Barderas and Benito-Peña)

The Yin-Yang biopanning method points out the probability of using crude antigens to isolate monoclonal antibodies with the phage display technique's help. (Shukra et al., 2014) Before using the phage display technique, animals are mainly used for synthetic antibody production, but this method of producing synthetic antibodies is expensive and time-consuming compared to the phage display technique. (Lim, 2019) Another advantage is that the phage display technique produces monoclonal antibodies with which human antibodies can be bound. (Hentrich et al., 2018)

The application of monoclonal antibodies to treat diseases caused by the virus has previously been studied, and specific monoclonal antibodies got approval for their application on humans. For example, ProteoGenix company inaugurated the detection of the antibody with enhanced therapeutic activity was done by selecting the library of naïve human antibodies (scFv, Lieb-SFMAX™, IgG, Fab) or library of human antibodies isolated from plasma of patients which become immune to COVID-19 with the help of bacteriophage display method. (Frenzel, 2017) It shows that the detection of an antibody with enhanced therapeutic activity is elementary.

There are two methods adopted by bacteriophages to reduce the death rate due to the pandemic of Covid-19. 1st method is that bacteriophages reduce the bacterial count by killing the bacteria present in the patient's respiratory system. 2nd method is the bacteriophage display technique used for producing synthetic anti--SARS-CoV-2 antibodies. (Dibo, 2019)Sequences of clinical trials are suggested using bacteriophages (phage cocktail), which kill all the major species involved in respiratory disorder, and by applying phage display technique for manufacturing synthetic antibodies that control the growth of SARS-CoV-2 at initial phases of infection.

Proposed Mechanisms for Anti-viral Activity of Bacteriophages
Inactivation of NF-κB by Bacteriophages during Viral Infection:

Bacteriophages present in the human body frequently travel from the gut to different body organs and tissues, including lungs, via transcytosis. It is estimated that 3×10^{10} bacteriophages move through the human body via transcytosis. (Wangersky and Lotka-Volterra, 1978) This constant flow of phages is supposed to be responsible for protecting against viruses. NF-κB regulates the expression of genes associated with immune response. Viruses replicate and multiply inside the bacterial host and evade cellular mechanism for eradicating viral infections by developing the strategies to use NF-κB signaling. The stimulation of NF-κB signaling is required to control several diseases caused by a virus, as shown in Figure 2.

As described earlier, phage therapy exhibits the capability of producing a vigorous immunological reaction against viruses. (Maslov and Sneppen, 2017) Irrespective of other viruses, phages against HSV (HSV-1 T4) do not involve the stimulation of NF-κB in epithelial and endothelial cells of humans. Moreover, if these cells are incubated with HSV-1 T4 phage, then the action of NF-κB is reduced and even wholly ended. According to a study, stimulation of NF-κB is entirely limited by phages against staphylococcus. (Eriksen et al., 2020) But this strategy of limiting stimulation of NF-κB is unrelated to its antibacterial activity. According to research conducted by Zhang et al., phage hinders HSV stimulated the activity of NF-κB. It is concluded from a review article regarding the available information that bacteriophages inhibit replication of viruses that infect eukaryotes inside the body and lab. This mechanism of phages to control viruses is necessary to understand. (Prazak et al., 2020)

There are seven transcriptional factors in the family of NF-κB, which are mainly involved in controlling the cellular response to inflammation and stress by regulating genes' expression (Rajnovic et al., 2019). Besides this, NF-κB is engaged in facilitating the apoptosis (programmed cell death) mechanism. Dimeric forms of transcriptional factors of NF-κB, such as present in the Rel family, possess transcription activation domain. (Barlow et al., 2020) Contrary to it, homodimeric conditions such as present in p52 and p50 do not include the transcription activation domain. The activity of NF-κB is controlled in a particular type of cell and towards a specific stimulus. In the case of viruses that infect eukaryotes, a particular virus signal attaches to specific receptors present on the section, leading to activation of IKK (IκB kinase).

IκB kinase performs phosphorylation of $I_k B\alpha$ (NF-κB inhibitor). After phosphorylation, $I_k B\alpha$ degrades by enzymes present in the proteasome. At the same time, NF-κB attaches to co-activators after entering the nucleus to stimulate the cell machinery involved in gene expression. (Dufour et al., 2019) As a result, Nk-κB is stimulated. Conversely, this Nk-κB activation mechanism has interfered with the protective functioning of phages. Phages hinder IkBα phosphorylation, which down-regulates the stimulation of NF-κB. As a result, the NF-κB activation mechanism is stopped (Górski et al.,

2019). Thus, a virus that infects eukaryotes is no more capable of activating transcription of the virus's genome.

Stimulation of Anti-Inflammatory Activity by Bacteriophages

Besides regulating NF-κB, bacteriophages also control other cellular mechanisms to perform protective functions. It is evaluated in a current study that the means of a cell are affected by A5/80 and T4 phage. It implies that phage therapy of cells by using any bacteriophage causes HSPA1 genes to overexpress. HSPA1 gene expresses and produces HSPA1 (heat shock 1A) protein of size 70kDa. It is also known as Hsp72. Many cell functions are performed by Hsp72, such as synthesis of protein, folding, and translocation. Moreover, Hsp72 protects the cell when it suffers from stress conditions like infection caused by a virus. (Górski et al., 2019)

In a study, an experiment shows that when T4 phage is applied on epithelial cells of human lungs suffering from an infection of Adv (human adenovirus), then survival of infected cells was observed during and after incubation. T4 phage demonstrated protective activity even when cells are pre-incubated with it. It is recognized that SARS-CoV-2 and SARS-CoV induce apoptosis, and consequently, deficiency of white blood cells (lymphocytopenia) has occurred. However, after harvesting and culturing human bronchi epithelial cells with bacteriophages in the lab, decreased apoptosis is seen. (Sharma et al., 2019)

A study demonstrates that the TLR10 gene is expressed by incubating with A5/80 bacteriophage. Among TLRs (toll-like receptors), the TLR10 gene is distinctive because it stimulates anti-inflammatory activity during the virus's infection. A5/80 phage tends to enhance IL-2 (inter- leaking-2) gene expression. Then, IL-2 boosts NK (natural killer) cell activity and facilitates the body to execute the anti-viral activity (Strydom et al., 2019).

T4 phage functions to activate the TLR2 gene together with the TLR10 gene after incubation. TLR2 exhibits specific property to identify the common capsid (protein coat) of the virus and stimulate the early immune response against the virus. The information mentioned above and data related to bacteriophages probably could pave the way to use bacteriophages to treat COVID-19.

Experiment for Bacteriophage Therapy—Bacteriophages as Prey

The main species of bacteria that are familiar to cause respiratory failures could minimize the aerosol application of bacteriophages in which they inhibit bacteria's growth rate. (Secor et al., 2015) This could have happened in a self-activating manner, same as ecological prey-predator order. If the bacterial population has already grown remarkably, bacteriophages' exponential growth should be needed for a fast clearance. Kill the-Winner population model, or Volterra can explain the relationship. Nebulized bacteriophages could cure pneumonia, and evidence available in the literature. (Reardon, 2019) Bacteriophages that are administered prophylactically minimize the bacterial load in the lungs and refer to ventilator-associated pneumonia; it enhanced the survival of antibiotic-resistant *S. aureus* infected animals (Giamarellos-Bourboulis et al., 2020). Screening methods can quickly identify the bacteria that cause respiratory problems and the specific species of bacteriophages that prey. In this way, selecting bacteriophages and identifying their target bacteria can become easy or quick.

During the clinical trials, (1) A group with a high probability of bacterial infections must be chosen. (2) Most effective in reducing bacterial population growth and targeting maximum bacteria, it should be ensured when selecting bacteriophages. (3) The adaptive or innate system of the patient is not affected by the bacteriophages. (4) Antibodies against bacteriophages do not already exist in the human body and do not develop to clear out bacteriophages before the bacteriophage-mediated killing of SARS-CoV-2. As compared with antibiotic treatment, we know that in bacteriophage therapy in case of pneumonia, the rapid bacterial lysis by bacteriophages in vivo causes no increase in the inflammatory response. It seemed to have positive effects on the patient's immune system, and it's a favorable finding. (5) According to the co-evolutionary method mentioned, bacterial species may be developed resistance against bacteriophage. It's another problem that could be a risk. But it's not a big deal and less severe than the pain of antibiotic resistance because the bacteriophage would only minimize the effectiveness of one bacteriophage, and there is also a possibility for phage that adapting to reduce any opposition to it. (6) There is no chance that the bacteriophage may harm any beneficial bacterial species because phages are so specific to their target species, but it still needs to be verified through clinical trials. There is also a point to be noted that the decrease in bacterial growth in a critical time gives the patient enough time to recover from the infection of Covid-19.

Reduction of Bacterial Growth Rate

Slow-going or lesser antibiotics response may be as expected. This may be the low diffusion rate and antibiotic-resistant strains in that domain because of bacterial biofilm formation. In some cases, the attacking of antibiotics into target tissues depends on the tissue type shown for lungs in tuberculosis scenarios. It has been revealed that in a patient's lungs, the sites of mycobacterial infection have poor vascularization and complex structures that block drug administration because it is elusive and hard to treat the disease sites. It is leading to suboptimal concentrations further. Due to their potential use for bacteriophages (undertake the patient's respiratory system indifferently and action on antibiotics as well) to minimize the patient's rate of mortality caused by SARS-CoV-2 virus.

In the hospitals or clinics which deal with Covid-19, antibiotics' intensive use can lead to further bacterial resistance. Using bacteriophages could ease this issue. Concerning post-Covid-19, the use of bacteriophages could also elucidate this problem.

Synthetic Antiviral Antibodies uses Minimize Viral Load

During the clinical trials, a presumption needs to be met in the second approach to work.   (1) High viral load and a bad prognosis (age >80) have to be chosen by cohort; (2) the selection of exact antibody that performs nothing in the body of a human but attacking the virus epitope; (3) Failure of the immune system should not cause by antibody (anaphylactic shock or an allergic reaction); (4) the frequency and dose should be quantitatively designed; and (5) the transportation system should be work accurately.

Knowledge Gaps

Literature studies will become essential to check possible known interactions before choosing the contender bacteriophages. For example, it has been shown that when bacteria are exposed to their specific bacteriophages, biofilm produced by some bacteria could create difficulties for Covid-19 patients in developing treatment methods. Some

21

bacteriophages can live inside the host without harming them while mostly kills their bacterial host. The present study provides many precautions to be followed carefully. For a while, in Covid-19 patients with severe respiratory failure, complex immune deregulation has been observed.

Conclusion

Bacteriophages can be used for treatment because they can be prepared cheaply and quickly when it is probably to prove experimental. Some production values may be shown by antibody production from phage display techniques, but it should be easy or straightforward due to current development. Moreover, bacteriophages can be easy to store and transport. SARS-CoV-2 prevalence is diminished by bacteriophages, especially in the patients affected by high viral load and bacterial infection of secondary type because they can be an experimental tool. There are no significant side effects, so it plays a vital role in saving lives. The beauty of nature showed us the mini creature that may be harmful but influential in the other aspects.

Acknowledgment:

I acknowledged all the authors for their contribution to this manuscript

Conflict of Interest:

All the authors have no conflict of interest.

References

Sung, J.J.Y., Will the SARS epidemic recur?, Sev. Acute. Respir. Syndr., 2004, vol. ,pp. 251–254.

Cevik, M., Bamford, C., and Ho, A., COVID-19 pandemic—A focused review for clinicians, *Clin. Microbiol. Infect.*, 2020, vol. 26, pp. 842-847.

Huang, C., Wang, Y., and Li, X., et al., Clinical features of pxxatients infected with 2019 novel coronavirus in Wuhan, China, *Lancet*, 2020, vol. 395, pp. 497–506.

Tay, M.Z., Poh, C.M., and Ré nia, L., et al, The trinity of COVID-19: Immunity, inflammation, and intervention, *Nat. Rev. Immunol.*, 2020, pp. 1–12.

Shi, Z., and Gewirtz, A., Together forever: Bacterial–viral interactions in infection and immunity, *Viruses*, 2018, vol. 10, pp. 122.

Stiasny, K., Aberle, J.H., and Keller, M., et al., Age affects quantity but not quality of antibody responses after vaccination with an inactivated flavivirus vaccine against tick-borne encephalitis, *PLoS One*, 2012, vol. 7, pp. e34145.

Ventura, MT., Casciaro, M., and Gangemi, S., et al., Immunosenescence in aging: Between immune cells depletion and cytokines up-regulation, *Clin. Mol. Allergy.*, 2017, vol 15, pp. 21.

Grijalva, C.G., Griffin, M.R., and Edwards, K.M., et al., The role of influenza and parainfluenza infections in nasopharyngeal pneumococcal acquisition among young children, *Clin. Infect. Dis.*, 2014, vol. 58 pp. 1369–1376.

Butler, J.C., and Schuchat, A., Epidemiology of pneumococcal infections in the elderly, *Drugs Aging.*, 1999, vol. 15, pp. 11–19.

Almand, E.A., Moore, M.D., and Jaykus, L.A., Virus-bacteria interactions: An emerging topic in human infection, *Viruses*, 2017, vol. 9, pp. 58.

Bosch, A.A.T.M., Biesbroek, G., and Trzcinski, K., et al., Viral and bacterial interactions in the upper respiratory tract, *PLoS Pathol.*, 2013, vol. 9, pp. e1003057.

Zhou, F., Yu, T., and Du, R., et al., Clinical course and risk factors for mortality of adult inpatients with COVID-19 in Wuhan, China: A retrospective cohort study, *Lancet,* 2020, vol. 395, pp. 1054–1062.

Dagur, H.S., Genome organization of Covid-19 and emerging severe acute respiratory syndrome Covid-19 outbreak: A pandemic, Eurasian J. Med. Oncol., 2020, vol.4, pp. 107–15.

Langan, K.M., Kotsimbos, T., and Peleg, A.Y., Managing *Pseudo- monas aeruginosa* respiratory infections in cystic fibrosis, *Curr. Opin. Infect. Dis.*, 2015, vol. 28, pp. 547–556.

Seki, M., Higashiyama, Y., and Tomono, K., et al., Acute infection with influenza virus enhances susceptibility to fatal pneumonia following *Streptococcus pneumoniae* infection in mice with chronic pulmonary colonization with *Pseudo- monas aeruginosa, Clin. Exp. Immunol.,* 2004, vol. 137, pp. 35–40.

Radetsky, P., *The Invisible Invaders: Viruses and the Scientists who Pursue Them*, Boston: Back Bay Books, 1994.

Al-Shayeb, B., Sachdeva, R., and Chen, L-X., et al., Clades of huge phages from across Earth's ecosystems, *Nature.* 2020, vol. 578, pp. 425–431.

Shkoporov, A.N., Hill, C., Bacteriophages of the human gut: The "Known Unknown" of the microbiome, *Cell Host Microbe*, 2019, vol. 25, pp. 195–209.

Koskella, B., and Meaden, S., Understanding bacteriophage specificity in natural microbial communities, *Viruses*, 2013, vol. 5, pp. 806–823.

Mueller, L., The red queen hypothesis, in *Conceptual Breakthroughs in Evolutionary Ecology,* Dulberger A, Avise J; eds. Cambridge, MA: Elsevier, Academic Press, 2020, pp. 85–86.

Papkou, A., Guzella, T., and Yang, W., et al., The genomic basis of Red Queen dynamics during rapid reciprocal host–pathogen coevolution, *Proc. Natl. Acad. Sci.*, 2019, vol. 116, pp. 923–928.

Willing, B., Russell, S., and Finlay, B., Shifting the balance: Antibiotic effects on host–microbiota mutualism, *Nat. Rev. Microbiol.*, 2011, vol. 9, pp. 233–243.

Salyers, A., The problem of antibiotic resistance, *Ann. Rev. Microbiol.*, 2003.

Aslam, B., Wang, W., and Arshad, M.I., et al., Antibiotic resistance: A rundown of a global crisis, *Infect. Drug Resist.,* 2018, vol. 11, pp. 1645–1658.

Hsu, J., How covid-19 is accelerating the threat of antimicrobial resistance, *BMJ*, 2020, pp. 369.

Czaplewski, L., Bax, R., and Clokie, M., et al., Alternatives to antibiotics-a pipeline portfolio review, *Lancet Infect. Dis.*, 2016, vol. 16, pp. 239–251.

Blanco-Picazo, P., Ferna´ndez-Orth, D., and Brown-Jaque, M., et al., Unravelling the consequences of the bacteriophages in human samples, *Sci. Rep.*, 2020, vol. 10, pp. 6737.

Nale, J.Y., Redgwell, T.A., and Millard, A., et al., Efficacy of an optimised bacteriophage cocktail to clear *Clostridium difficile* in a batch fermentation model. Antibiotics, 2018, vol. 7, pp. 13.

Nir-Paz, R., Gelman, D., and Khouri, A., et al., Successful treatment of antibiotic-resistant, poly-microbial bone infection with bacteriophages and antibiotics combination, *Clin. Infect. Dis.*, 2019, vol. 69, pp. 2015–2018.

Cafora, M., Deflorian, G., and Forti, F., et al., Phage therapy against *Pseudomonas aeruginosa* infections in a cystic fibrosis zebrafish model, *Sci. Rep.*, 2019, vol. 9, pp. 1–10

Peng, H., Borg, R.E., and Dow, L.P., et al., Controlled phage therapy by photothermal ablation of specific bacterial species using gold nanorods targeted by chimeric phages, *Proc. Natl. Acad. Sci. U S A.*, 2020, vol. 117, pp. 1951–1961.

Barderas, R., and Benito-Peña, E., The 2018 Nobel Prize in Chemistry: Phage display of peptides and antibodies, *Anal. Bioanal. Chem.*, 2019, vol. 411, pp. 2475–2479.

Shukra, A.M., Sridevi, N.V., Dev, and Chandran., et al., Production of recombinant antibodies using bacteriophages, *Eur. J. Microbiol. Immunol.*, 2014, vol. 4, pp. 91–98.

Lim, C.C., Woo, P.C.Y., and Lim, T.S., Development of a phage display panning strategy utilizing crude antigens: Isolation of MERS-CoV nucleoprotein human antibodies, *Sci. Rep.,* 2019, vol. 9, pp. 6088.

Hentrich, C., Ylera, F., and Frisch, C., et al., Monoclonal antibody generation by phage display, in *Handbook of Immunoassay Technologies,*

Vashist S.K., Luony J.H.T., Eds., Cambridge, MA: Elsevier, Academic Press, 2018, pp. 47–80.

Frenzel, A., Kügler, J., and Helmsing, S., et al., Designing human antibodies by phage display, *Transfus. Med. Hemother.*, 2017, vol. 44, pp. 312–318.

Dibo, M., Battocchio, E.C., Dos, Santos, and Souza, L.M., et al., Antibody therapy for the control of viral diseases: An update, Curr. Pharm. Biotechnol., 2019, vol. 20, pp. 1108–1121.

Wangersky, PJ., Lotka-Volterra, Population models. *Ann. Rev. Ecol. Syst.*, 1978. Vol. 9, pp. 189–218.

Maslov, S., and Sneppen, K., Population cycles and species diversity in dynamic Kill-the-Winner model of microbial ecosystems, *Sci. Rep.,* 2017, vol. 7, pp. 39642.

Eriksen, R.S., Mitarai, N., and Sneppen, K., Sustainability of spatially distributed bacteria-phage systems, *Sci. Rep.*, 2020, vol. 10, pp. 3154.

Prazak, J., Valente, L., and Iten, M., et al., Nebulized bacteriophages for prophylaxis of experimental ventilator-associated pneumonia due to methicillin-resistant *Staphylococcus aureus. Crit Care Med.,* 2020.

Rajnovic, D., Muñoz-Berbel, X., and Mas, J., Fast phage detection and quantification: An optical density-based approach, *PLoS One*, 2019, vol. 14, pp. e0216292.

Barlow, J.T., Bogatyrev, S.R., and Ismagilov, R.F., A quantitative sequencing framework for absolute abundance measurements of mucosal and lumenal microbial communities, *Nature communications,* 2020, vol. 11, pp. 1-13.

Dufour, N., Delattre, R., and Chevallereau, A., et al., Phage therapy of pneumonia is not associated with an overstimulation of the inflammatory response compared to antibiotic treatment in mice, *Antimicrob. Agents Chemother.,* 2019, vol. 63, pp. e00379-19.

Górski, A., Międzybrodzki, R., and Jończyk-Matysiak, E., et al., Phage-specific diverse effects of bacterial viruses on the immune system, *Future Microbiol.,* 2019, vol. 14, pp. 1171–1174.

Sharma, D., Misba, L., and Khan, A.U., Antibiotics versus biofilm: An emerging battleground in microbial communities, *Antimicrob. Resist. Infect. Control.,* 2019, vol. 8, pp. 76.

Strydom, N., Gupta, S.V., Fox W.S, et al., Tuberculosis drugs' distribution and emergence of resistance in patient's lung lesions: A mechanistic model and tool for regimen and dose optimization, *PLoS Med.,* 2019, vol. 16, pp. e1002773.

Secor, P.R., Sweere, J.M., and Michaels, L.A., et al., Filamentous bacteriophage promote biofilm assembly and function, *Cell Host Microbe,* 2015, vol. 18, pp. 549–559.

Reardon, S., Virus tricks the immune system into ignoring bacterial infections, *Nature,* 2019.

Giamarellos-Bourboulis, E.J., Netea, M.G., and Rovina, N., et al., Complex immune dysregulation in COVID-19 patients with severe respiratory failure, *Cell Host Microbe,* 2020.

Abedon, S. T., Kuhl, S. J., Blasdel, B. G., Kutter, E. M., Abedon, S. T., Kuhl, S. J., Blasdel, B. G., & Martin, E. (2011). *Phage treatment of human infections a n d e s i o s c i e n c e o. 7081.* https://doi.org/10.4161/bact.1.2.15845

Abedon, S. T., & Thomas-abedon, C. (2010). *Phage Therapy Pharmacology.* 28–47.

Aminov, R. I., Otto, M., & Sommer, A. (2010). *A brief history of the antibiotic era : lessons learned and challenges for the future. 1*(December), 1–7. https://doi.org/10.3389/fmicb.2010.00134

Arndt, D., Grant, J. R., Marcu, A., Sajed, T., Pon, A., Liang, Y., & Wishart, D. S. (2016). *PHASTER : a better , faster version of the PHAST phage search tool. 44*(May), 16–21. https://doi.org/10.1093/nar/gkw387

Bonilla, N., Rojas, M. I., Netto, G., Cruz, F., Hung, S., Rohwer, F., & Barr, J. J. (2016). *Phage on tap – a quick and efficient protocol for the preparation of bacteriophage laboratory stocks.* https://doi.org/10.7717/peerj.2261

Caprinos, E. (2008). *An alternative method for.* 299–306.

Chan, B. K., Abedon, S. T., & Loc-carrillo, C. (2013). *Phage cocktails and the future of phage therapy.* 769–783.

Chaudhry, W. N., Haq, I. U., Andleeb, S., & Qadri, I. (2013). *Characterization of a virulent bacteriophage LK1 speci fi c for Citrobacter freundii isolated from sewage water.* 1–11. https://doi.org/10.1002/jobm.201200710

Drulis-kawa, Z., Majkowska-skrobek, G., Maciejewska, B., Delattre, A., & Lavigne, R. (2012). *Learning from Bacteriophages - Advantages and Limitations of Phage and Phage-Encoded Protein Applications. i,* 699–722.

Endersen, L., Mahony, J. O., Hill, C., Ross, R. P., Mcauliffe, O., & Coffey, A. (2014). *Phage Therapy in the Food Industry.* https://doi.org/10.1146/annurev-food-030713-092415

Fadlallah, A., Chelala, E., & Legeais, J. (2015). *Corneal Infection Therapy with*

Topical Bacteriophage Administration. 8505, 167–168.

Gill, J. J., & Hyman, P. (2010). *Phage Choice , Isolation , and Preparation for Phage Therapy.* 2–14.

Golkar, Z., Bagasra, O., & Pace, D. G. (n.d.). *Review Article Bacteriophage therapy : a potential solution for the antibiotic resistance crisis.* https://doi.org/10.3855/jidc.3573

Klumpp, J., Lavigne, R., & Loessner, M. J. (2010). *The SPO1-related bacteriophages.* 1547–1561. https://doi.org/10.1007/s00705-010-0783-0

Kutter, E. M., Kuhl, S. J., & Abedon, S. T. (2015). *Re-establishing a place for phage therapy in western medicine. 10*, 685–688.

Lu, T. K., & Koeris, M. S. (2011). The next generation of bacteriophage therapy. *Current Opinion in Microbiology, 14*(5), 524–531. https://doi.org/10.1016/j.mib.2011.07.028

Merrill, B. D., Ward, A. T., Grose, J. H., & Hope, S. (2016). Software-based analysis of bacteriophage genomes , physical ends , and packaging strategies. *BMC Genomics*, 1–16. https://doi.org/10.1186/s12864-016-3018-2

Meyer, J. R., Flores, C. O., Weitz, J. S., Valverde, S., Sullivan, M. B., & Hochberg, M. E. (2013). *Phage – bacteria infection networks. 21*(2). https://doi.org/10.1016/j.tim.2012.11.003

Miedzybrodzki, R., Fortuna, W., Weber-Dabrowska, B., & Górski, A. (2007). Phage therapy of staphylococcal infections (including MRSA) may be less expensive than antibiotic treatment. *Postepy Higieny i Medycyny Doświadczalnej (Online), 61*, 461–465. https://doi.org/495359 [pii]

Pelfrene, E., Willebrand, E., Sanches, A. C., Sebris, Z., & Cavaleri, M. (2017). *Bacteriophage therapy : a regulatory perspective. April 2016*, 2071–2074. https://doi.org/10.1093/jac/dkw083

Pirnay, J., Blasdel, B. G., Bretaudeau, L., Buckling, A., Chanishvili, N., Clark, J. R., & Corte-real, S. (2015). *Quality and Safety Requirements for Sustainable Phage Therapy Products.* 2173–2179. https://doi.org/10.1007/s11095-014-1617-7

Pirnay, J., Vos, D. De, Verbeken, G., Merabishvili, M., Chanishvili, N., Vaneechoutte, M., & Zizi, M. (2011). *The Phage Therapy Paradigm : Prêt-à-Porter or Sur-mesure?* 934–937. https://doi.org/10.1007/s11095-010-0313-5

Plaza, N., Castillo, D., Pérez-reytor, D., Higuera, G., García, K., & Bastías, R. (2018). *Bacteriophages in the control of pathogenic vibrios. 31*, 24–33. https://doi.org/10.1016/j.ejbt.2017.10.012

Prazak, J., Iten, M., Cameron, D. R., Save, J., Grandgirard, D., Resch, G., Goepfert, C., Leib, S. L., Takala, J., Jakob, S. M., Que, Y. A., & Haenggi, M. (2019). Bacteriophages improve outcomes in experimental staphylococcus aureus ventilator-associated pneumonia. *American Journal of Respiratory and Critical Care Medicine, 200*(9), 1126–1133. https://doi.org/10.1164/rccm.201812-2372OC

Rakonjac, J., & Bennett, N. J. (2009). *Filamentous Bacteriophage : Biology , Phage Display and Nanotechnology Applications.* 51–76.

Ryan, E. M., Alkawareek, M. Y., Donnelly, R. F., Gilmore, B. F., & Gilmore, C. B. F. (2012). *IMMUNOLOGY & MEDICAL MICROBIOLOGY.* https://doi.org/10.1111/j.1574-695X.2012.00977.x

Ryan, E. M., Gorman, S. P., Donnelly, R. F., & Gilmore, B. F. (2011). *Recent advances in bacteriophage therapy : how delivery routes , formulation , concentration and timing influence the success of phage therapy.* 1253–1264. https://doi.org/10.1111/j.2042-7158.2011.01324.x

Summers, W. C. (2010). *Cholera and Plague in India: The Bacteriophage*

Inquiry of 1927-193 6 Downloaded from. 48, 275–301. https://sites.ualberta.ca/~pukatzki/labpage/Lab_News/Entries/2010/11/14_P hage_Therapy_files/The Bacteriophage Inquiry.pdf

Valleys, D., Wei, S. T. S., & Higgins, C. M. (2015). *Genetic signatures indicate widespread antibiotic resistance and phage infection in microbial communities of the McMurdo.* https://doi.org/10.1007/s00300-015-1649-4

Figures

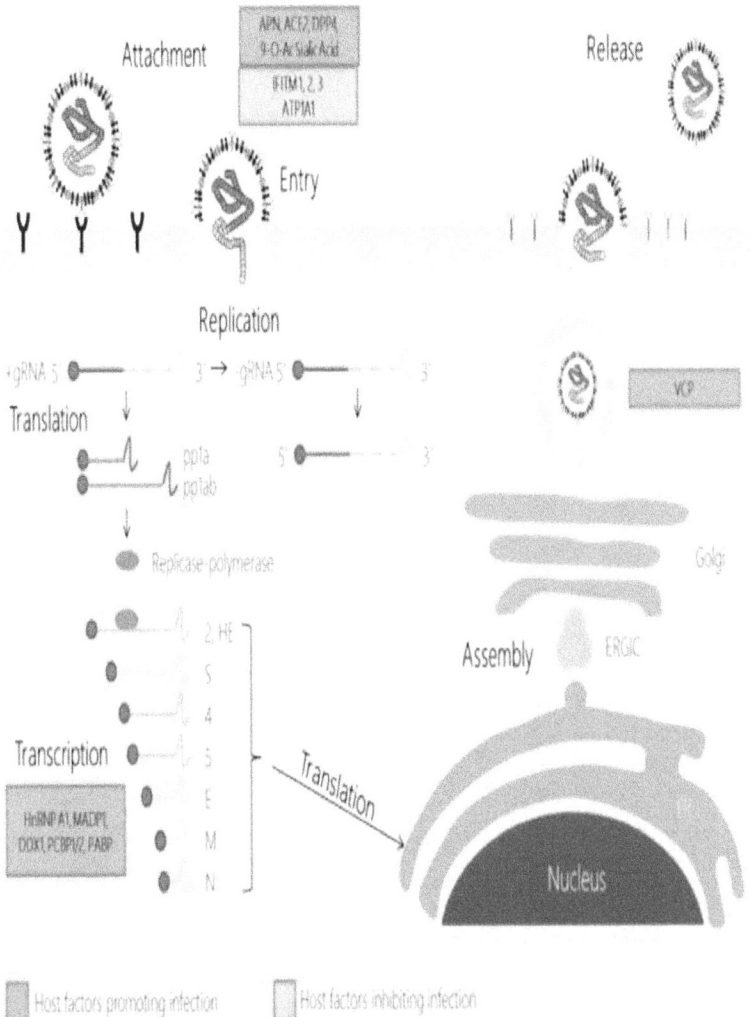

FIGURE 1: Schematic representation of coronavirus replication cycle (image from Xinyi et al., *Diseases* 4 (3) (2016): 26; https://www.ncbi.

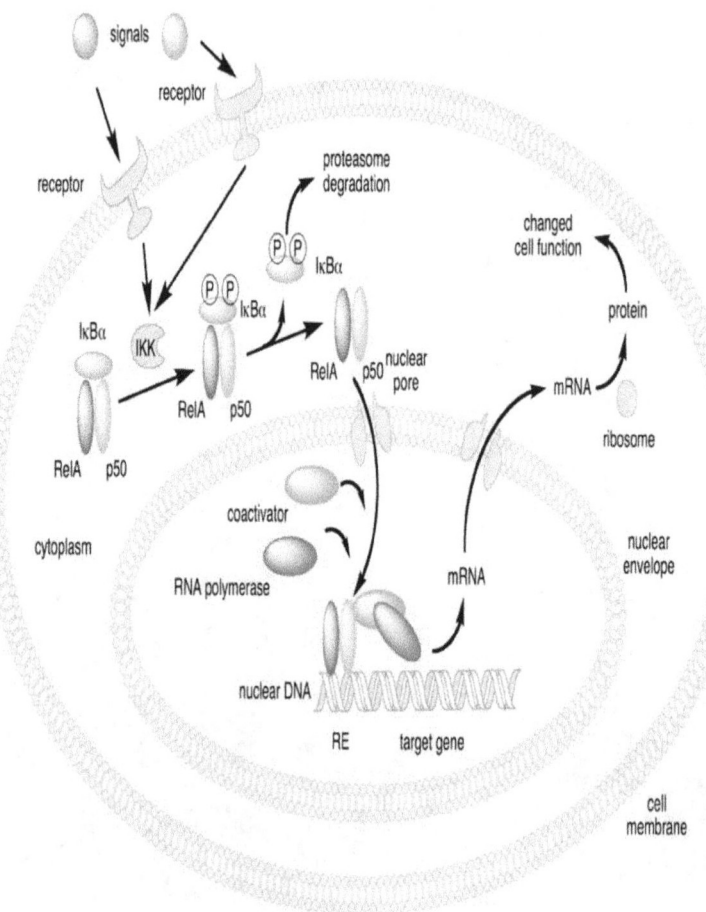

F<small>IGURE</small> 2: Mechanism of phage action in the bacterial cell (Wikimedia Commons. Retrieved 17:38, August 29, 2020, from https://commons. wikimedia.org/w/index.php?titleFile: NFKB_mechanism_of_action.png&oldid232074767).

Publisher: Eliva Press SRL

Email: info@elivapress.com

www.ingramcontent.com/pod-product-compliance
Lightning Source LLC
Chambersburg PA
CBHW051301170526
45165CB00004B/1806